COPD DIET COOKBOOK: FOR NEWLY DIAGNOSED

Say goodbye to copd pain with our special delicious recipes to conquer and restoring your healthy,+28day meal plan to balance wellness.

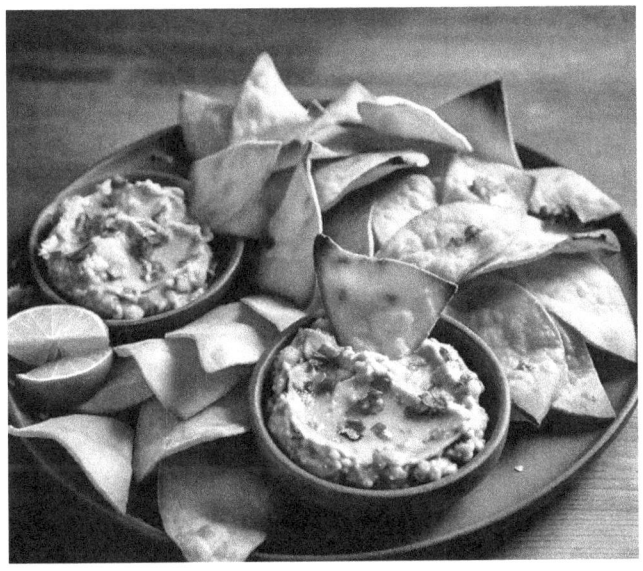

Dr. Jerry Cole

Copyright © 2024 Dr. Jerry Cole
Allright Reserved

No part of this publication may be reproduce, stored in a retrieval system, or transmitted in any form or by any means, electronic, mechanical, photocopying, recording or otherwise, without the prior permission of the copyright owner.

TABLE OF CONTENT

INTRODUCTION... 6
COPD: WHAT IS IT?... 8
WHAT SIGNS AND CAUSES CORRESPOND WITH COPD?... 9
ADVANTAGES OF COPD... 11
FOOD TO AVOID IN COPD..................................... 14
FOODS TO INCLUDE IN COPD................................ 17
GETTING STARTED FOR COPD NEWLY DIAGNOSED 21
COOKING WITH COPD NEWLY DIAGNOSIS............. 25
BREAKFAST RECIPES... 30
Oatmeal with Berries:... 30
Avocado Toast with Egg:...................................... 31
Greek Yogurt Parfait:... 32
Spinach and Tomato Omelette:............................. 34
Smoothie with Protein:... 35
LUNCH RECIPES... 37
Quinoa Salad with Grilled Chicken:....................... 37
Turkey and Avocado Wrap:................................... 39
Salmon and Quinoa Bowl:..................................... 40
Vegetable and Lentil Soup:................................... 42
Caprese Salad with Whole Grain Bread:................ 43
DINNER RECIPES... 45
Baked Lemon Herb Chicken with Roasted Vegetables:.. 45
Vegetable Stir-Fry with Tofu:................................ 47
Salmon with Asparagus and Lemon Dill Sauce:..... 49

Turkey and Vegetable Skillet:................................. 51

Vegetable and Bean Soup:..................................... 53

6. Taste and adjust seasoning if needed. Serve hot, optionally garnished with freshly chopped parsley.... 55

APPETIZER RECIPES...55

Vegetable Crudité with Hummus:............................ 55

Caprese Skewers:...57

Guacamole with Baked Tortilla Chips:...................... 58

Smoked Salmon Cucumber Bites:............................60

Stuffed Mushrooms:..61

HEALTHY RECIPES... 63

Salmon Salad with Lemon-Dill Dressing:..................63

Quinoa and Black Bean Salad:................................65

Turkey and Vegetable Stir-Fry:................................67

Spinach and Chickpea Curry:.................................. 69

Vegetable and Lentil Soup:.....................................72

SNACKS AND DESSERT RECIPES............................74

SNACKS:.. 74

Yogurt with Berries and Almonds:...........................74

Vegetable Sticks with Hummus:.............................. 75

Apple Slices with Peanut Butter:............................. 76

Cottage Cheese with Pineapple:............................. 77

Trail Mix:...77

DESSERTS:.. 78

Frozen Yogurt Bark:... 79

Banana Oatmeal Cookies:...................................... 80

Chia Seed Pudding:..81

Baked Apples with Cinnamon and Walnuts:............83

Frozen Banana Bites: 85
28DAY MEAL PLAN 86
Day 1: 86
Day 2: 87
Day 3: 88
Day 4: 89
Day 5: 90
Day 6: 90
Day 7: 91
Day 8: 92
Day 9: 92
Day 10: 93
Day 11: 94
Day 12: 95
Day 13: 96
Day 14: 96
Day 15: 97
Day 16: 98
Day 17: 99
Day 18: 100
Day 19: 100
Day 20: 101
Day 21: 102
Day 22: 103
Day 23: 104
Day 24: 104
Day 25: 105
Day 26: 106

Day 27:..107
Day 28:..108
CONCLUSION..109
THE END..110

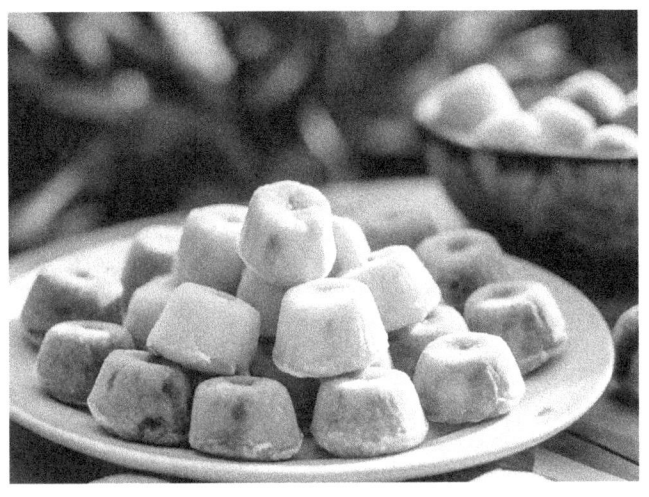

INTRODUCTION

"Welcome to your new breath of life! If you're newly diagnosed with Chronic Obstructive Pulmonary Disease (COPD), you may be feeling overwhelmed and unsure of where to start. But take a deep breath - you're not alone! This cookbook is here to guide you on a journey towards easier breathing, better health, and a more vibrant life.

With COPD, every bite counts. The right foods can help you breathe easier, reduce symptoms, and feel more energized. And that's exactly what this cookbook is all about - delicious, easy-to-make recipes that are gentle on your lungs and nourishing for your body.

In the following pages, you'll discover:

- How to identify and avoid trigger foods
- How to incorporate lung-friendly ingredients into your diet
- How to cook and meal prep with ease
- How to enjoy flavorful, nutritious meals that support your health

Take a deep breath, and let's get started on this journey together! With this cookbook, you'll be breathing easier and living better in no time."

This introduction aims to:

- Welcome and reassure the reader
- Emphasize the importance of diet in managing COPD
- Highlight the benefits of the cookbook
- Encourage the reader to start their journey towards better health and easier breathing.

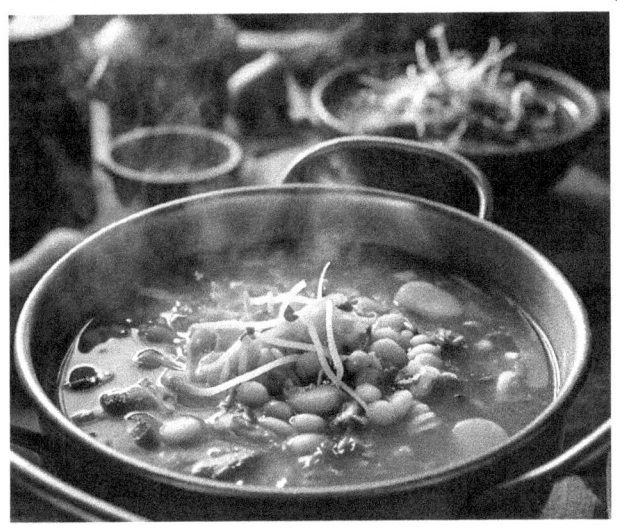

COPD: WHAT IS IT?

Chronic Obstructive Pulmonary Disease is referred to as COPD. It is a long-term inflammatory lung condition that obstructs lung airflow. Long-term exposure to irritating chemicals or particulate matter—most frequently from cigarette smoke—is the usual cause of this illness.

Coughing, wheezing, shortness of breath, and tightness in the chest are signs of COPD. With time, COPD can significantly impair breathing and cause consequences like heart issues and respiratory infections. Since the illness is progressive, it usually gets worse with time.

The goals of COPD treatment are to reduce symptoms, delay the course of the illness, and enhance quality of life. In severe situations, this may entail lung transplantation or surgery in addition to oxygen therapy, pulmonary rehabilitation, and medicines. Important efforts in controlling COPD include avoiding lung irritants and quitting smoking.

WHAT SIGNS AND CAUSES CORRESPOND WITH COPD?

Although the intensity of COPD symptoms varies, they often include:

Dyspnea, or shortness of breath, is frequently the first symptom to be recognized, particularly when engaging in strenuous exercise.
A chronic cough is one that lasts longer than usual and may produce clear, white, yellow, or greenish sputum.
Squeaky or whistling sound made during breathing is called wheezing.
Tightness in the chest: A constriction or discomfort in the chest.
Recurrent respiratory infections: Respiratory infections like pneumonia and bronchitis can become more common in people with COPD.
Fatigue: Having little energy or feeling exhausted, usually from breathing more deeply.
Regarding causes, prolonged exposure to lung irritants—most frequently, cigarette smoke—is the main risk factor for COPD.

Additional variables that may be involved in COPD include:

extended exposure to additional lung irritants, such as dust, chemical fumes, or air pollution.

Genetic factors: Individuals with a lack of alpha-1-antitrypsin protein may be more susceptible to developing COPD due to genetics.

Repeated respiratory infections: Having severe or recurrent respiratory infections as a child raises the chance of getting COPD in later life.

Occupational exposure: Working in jobs where there is a lot of dust, chemicals, or fumes can make you more likely to get COPD.

While smoking and COPD are frequently linked, it's vital to remember that not everyone with COPD smokes. Similar to how not everyone who smokes gets COPD, smoking is the main cause of the illness. Furthermore, COPD tends to progress slowly over many years, so symptoms could not show up until serious lung damage has taken place.

ADVANTAGES OF COPD

COPD has no inherent advantages because it is a progressive, chronic illness. Nonetheless, there are a few areas of COPD treatment and care where particular behaviors or methods can be advantageous for those who have the illness:

The single most essential thing you can do to slow down the advancement of COPD and enhance your general health is to stop smoking. Over time, stopping smoking can improve lung function, lessen symptoms, and cut down on the frequency of exacerbations, or flare-ups.

Pulmonary rehabilitation: People with COPD may benefit greatly from taking part in pulmonary rehabilitation programs. The goals of these programs are usually to improve lung function, lessen symptoms, and improve quality of life. They usually include fitness training, information, and support.

Medication: Although bronchodilators and inhaled corticosteroids are not able to treat COPD, they can help control symptoms and enhance lung function. These drugs can lessen dyspnea, lessen the frequency of exacerbations, and enhance general quality of life when used as directed.

Oxygen therapy: By increasing tissue oxygenation, lowering dyspnea, and enhancing exercise tolerance, supplementary oxygen therapy can be beneficial in cases of severe COPD with low blood oxygen levels.

Lifestyle adjustments: Changing one's diet, engaging in physical activity within reason, and limiting exposure to lung irritants (including secondhand smoke and air pollution) can all help control the symptoms of COPD and enhance general health.

Social support: Whether it comes from friends, family, or support organizations, having a strong social network can offer consolation, inspiration, and useful help in overcoming the difficulties of living with COPD.

Even though COPD presents many difficulties, managing the illness proactively can enhance quality of life, reduce symptoms, and improve overall health.

FOOD TO AVOID IN COPD

Maintaining a balanced diet is crucial for COPD patients in order to promote general health and wellbeing. People with COPD may benefit from minimizing or avoiding some meals and beverages that could increase symptoms or contribute to health difficulties, even though there are no certain items that need to be avoided totally. Here are a few broad recommendations:

High-Sodium Foods: Eating too much salt can exacerbate symptoms like dyspnea and cause fluid retention. Eat less or stay away from items high in sodium, such as processed meals, soups in cans, salty snacks, and fast food.

Foods that Produce Gas: Certain foods have the potential to produce gas and bloating, which can worsen stomach pain and make breathing more difficult. Broccoli, cabbage, onions, beans, and fizzy drinks are a few examples. Even though these meals are healthy, people might need to cut back on their consumption or find different ways to cook in order to produce less gas.

Heavy or Fatty Foods: Breathing becomes more difficult and bloating might occur after large, heavy meals. Eating foods high in fat can also cause weight gain, which puts stress on the respiratory system. Choose meals that are lighter and more well-balanced, with plenty of fruits, vegetables, whole grains, and lean proteins.

Caffeinated Beverages: Although most people may safely consume modest amounts of caffeine, consuming too much of these drinks—such as energy drinks, coffee, and tea—can lead to dehydration and disrupt sleep. For people with COPD, maintaining proper hydration is crucial, thus it's critical to balance coffee and water intake.

Alcoholic Beverages: When ingested in excess, alcohol can aggravate respiratory depression and interact negatively with several drugs. It can also cause respiratory depression. If alcohol is used at all, it should be done so in moderation. You should also be aware of any possible drug interactions with COPD drugs.

Foods That May Cause Allergies: People with COPD may also be allergic to or sensitive to certain foods, including dairy, gluten, or particular fruits and vegetables. After taking any particular food, be aware of any negative effects and seek medical advice if needed.

Overall, treating COPD and promoting general health depend on eating a well-balanced diet that contains a range of nutrient-dense foods. It's critical that people with COPD collaborate with a medical professional or registered dietitian to create a customized eating plan that satisfies their unique nutritional requirements and advances their lung health objectives.

FOODS TO INCLUDE IN COPD

Including foods high in nutrients in the diet can assist people with COPD stay healthy overall and effectively manage their symptoms. The following foods might be advantageous for those who have COPD:

Fruits and vegetables: Packed with fiber, antioxidants, vitamins, and minerals, these foods can boost the immune system and lower inflammation. Aim for a range of vibrant fruits and vegetables, including tomatoes, bell peppers, leafy greens, berries, and citrus fruits.

Lean Proteins: Include foods like fish, poultry, eggs, tofu, lentils, and nuts in your diet. Protein is necessary for the maintenance and regeneration of muscles, which helps assist respiratory muscles and general strength in COPD patients.

Whole Grains: To enhance fiber intake and offer long-lasting energy, go for whole grains rather than processed grains. Whole wheat bread, brown rice, quinoa, oats, and barley are a few examples.

Good Fats: Include foods high in healthy fats in your diet, such as avocados, nuts, seeds, olive oil, and fatty fish (like mackerel and salmon). Essential fatty acids are provided by healthy fats, which may also help lower inflammation.

Dairy or Dairy Alternatives: Calcium and vitamin D, which are crucial for bone health, can be found in dairy products and fortified dairy substitutes (such almond milk or soy milk). On the other hand, people who are intolerant to dairy or have sensitivities to it can choose lactose-free dairy products or other calcium-rich foods like leafy greens or fortified non-dairy milk.

Fluids: To help reduce mucus productions and avoid dehydration, it's critical for people with COPD to maintain adequate hydration. Make it a point to stay hydrated during the day by consuming lots of water, herbal teas, and broths. Drinks high in alcohol or caffeine, however, should be avoided as they might exacerbate dehydration.

Small, Frequently Spaced Meals: By avoiding bloating and discomfort, eating smaller, more frequent meals throughout the day may facilitate better breathing. For long-lasting energy, prioritize eating balanced meals that contain a mix of healthy fats, proteins, and carbs.

Anti-Inflammatory Foods: Several foods include anti-inflammatory qualities that may aid in the body's reduction of inflammation. Green tea, onions, garlic, ginger, and turmeric are a few examples. By consuming these foods, you may be able to control the symptoms of COPD.

Omega-3 Fatty Acids: Rich in fatty fish, flaxseeds, chia seeds, and walnuts, omega-3 fatty acids have anti-inflammatory qualities that may help people with COPD by lowering inflammation and enhancing lung function.

It's critical that people with COPD collaborate with a medical professional or registered dietitian to create a customized eating plan that satisfies their unique nutritional requirements and advances their lung health objectives.

GETTING STARTED FOR COPD NEWLY DIAGNOSED

Although receiving a COPD diagnosis might be upsetting, there are things you can do to manage the illness and enhance your quality of life. Here is a starting point guide to assist you:

Learn About COPD: Become knowledgeable about the causes, signs, and available treatments of COPD. Gaining knowledge about your illness can help you take control of your health and effectively manage your symptoms.

Give Up Smoking: The most crucial thing you can do to improve your lung health and slow the course of COPD is to give up smoking. To successfully stop smoking, get aid from medical specialists, programs for quitting, or support groups.

Adhere to Your Treatment Plan: Create a customized treatment plan that meets your needs by consulting closely with your healthcare provider. This could involve changing one's lifestyle, taking oxygen treatment, pulmonary rehabilitation, and medication. Remember to keep all of your regular appointments and take your meds as directed.

Participating in a pulmonary rehabilitation program is something you should think about doing. These programs provide instruction, support, and supervised fitness training to help you feel better overall, function better in your lungs, and lessen symptoms.

Remain Active: Engaging in regular physical activity can help you breathe better, build stronger muscles, and have more energy. Begin with mild workouts like swimming, cycling, or walking, and progressively raise your level of activity as tolerated.

Eat a Balanced Diet: Make sure your meals are full of entire grains, fruits, veggies, lean meats, and healthy fats. You can stay at a healthy weight, have energy, and boost your immune system with proper eating.

Keep Yourself Hydrated: To help maintain mucus thin and avoid dehydration, drink lots of fluids throughout the day. Drink at least eight glasses of water each day, and limit your intake of alcohol and caffeine.

Handle Stress: Since COPD can be a stressful condition, it's critical to learn appropriate coping mechanisms for tension and anxiety. Engage in relaxation exercises like yoga, tai chi, meditation, or deep breathing. You should also think about getting help from a therapist or support group.

Reduce Your Exposure to Lung Irritants: Reduce the amount of dust, chemicals, air pollution, and cigarette smoke that irritate your lungs. Discuss measures to lessen your exposure to environmental toxins at work with your employer.

Keep in Touch: Ask friends, family, and medical experts for assistance. Never be afraid to ask for assistance when you need it, and think about joining a COPD support group to get in touch with people who are in similar situations as you.

Recall that living with COPD is a lifetime journey, and that experiencing highs and lows is commonplace. Remember to take charge of your health, adhere to your treatment plan, and don't be afraid to ask for help when you need it. With the correct assistance and care, COPD can be effectively managed.

COOKING WITH COPD NEWLY DIAGNOSIS

Cooking can be difficult when you have COPD, but you can still enjoy making and eating scrumptious, nourishing meals with a few adjustments and tricks. The following advice will help you cook in comfort and safety:

Plan Ahead: To avoid stress and exhaustion, schedule your meals in advance. Think about making quick and easy meals that only need a little amount of time and work. To save time, consider convenience items like cooked grains or pre-cut vegetables.

Select Quick and Simple Recipes: Seek out recipes that are simple to make and call for a minimal number of steps. Convenient options that require less hands-on cooking time include sheet pan dinners, slow cooker dishes, and one-pot meals.

Use Kitchen Gadgets and Tools: Make cooking easier by making use of kitchen gadgets and tools. Invest in ergonomic kitchenware and appliances that will ease the strain on your hands and joints. Use a food processor or blender to chop vegetables or purée items.

Organize Your Kitchen: To improve cooking efficiency, keep your kitchen tidy and orderly. Use labels or clear containers to help you immediately identify ingredients and supplies, and keep frequently used things easily accessible.

Take Breaks: When cooking, pace yourself and stop as needed to refuel and regain your breath. If you feel faint or exhausted, take a seat, and pay attention to your body's signals so you don't overdo it.

Reduce Odors and Irritants: Try to reduce your exposure to strong smells and lung irritants since cooking fumes and odors might aggravate your COPD symptoms. To lessen indoor air pollution, try cooking using electric appliances rather than gas ones and use exhaust fans or open windows to ventilate your kitchen.

Remain Safe: To lower the possibility of mishaps and injuries, take safety precautions when cooking. When handling hot dishes, put on oven mitts or potholders and exercise caution near hot surfaces and sharp objects. For jobs requiring extra strength or coordination, think about asking a family member or caretaker for assistance.

Keep Hydrated: To stay hydrated and avoid dehydration when cooking, consume a lot of liquids. Especially if you're working in a hot or muggy area, keep a bottle of water close by and take frequent sips from it.

Simplify Cleanup: Line baking sheets with parchment paper or aluminum foil and use disposable cooking utensils to make cleanup easier. To make cleaning easier, ask family members for assistance or use a dishwasher.

Ask for Help: If you need help with household chores or meal preparation, don't be afraid to ask for it. Cooking with COPD can be made easier with the support and help of friends, family, and caregivers.

You can keep enjoying creating delectable meals while successfully treating COPD by paying attention to these suggestions and making changes as necessary. Pay attention to your body, put your health and safety first, and don't be afraid to ask for help when you need it.

BREAKFAST RECIPES

Oatmeal with Berries:

Ingredients:

1. 1/2 cup rolled oats
2. 1 cup water or milk (dairy or plant-based)
3. 1/4 cup mixed berries (blueberries, raspberries, strawberries)
4. 1 tablespoon honey or maple syrup (optional)
- Instructions:
    1. In a small saucepan, bring water or milk to a boil.
    2. Stir in rolled oats and reduce heat to

medium-low. Cook for 5-7 minutes, stirring occasionally, until oats are creamy.
3. Remove from heat and let it cool slightly.
4. Top with mixed berries and drizzle with honey or maple syrup if desired.

Avocado Toast with Egg:

- Ingredients:
    1. 1 slice whole grain bread
    2. 1/2 ripe avocado
    3. 1 egg
    4. Salt and pepper to taste
- Instructions:

1. Toast the bread until golden brown.
2. Mash the avocado and spread it on top of the toast.
3. Fry or poach the egg to your preference.
4. Place the cooked egg on top of the avocado toast.
5. Season with salt and pepper.

Greek Yogurt Parfait:

- Ingredients:
    1. 1/2 cup Greek yogurt
    2. 1/4 cup granola (choose low-sugar option)

3. 1/4 cup mixed fruits (such as bananas, berries, or sliced apples)
4. 1 tablespoon honey (optional)
- Instructions:
    1. In a glass or bowl, layer Greek yogurt, granola, and mixed fruits.
    2. Repeat the layers until all ingredients are used.
    3. Drizzle with honey if desired.

Spinach and Tomato Omelette:

- Ingredients:
    1. 2 eggs

2. 1/4 cup fresh spinach leaves
3. 1/4 cup diced tomatoes
4. 1 tablespoon olive oil
5. Salt and pepper to taste
- Instructions:
  1. In a bowl, beat the eggs and season with salt and pepper.
  2. Heat olive oil in a non-stick skillet over medium heat.
  3. Add spinach and tomatoes to the skillet and cook for 1-2 minutes until spinach wilts.
  4. Pour the beaten eggs over the spinach and tomatoes.
  5. Cook until the edges are set, then carefully flip the omelette and cook for another 1-2 minutes.
  6. Fold the omelette in half and serve hot.

Smoothie with Protein:

- Ingredients:
    1. 1/2 cup Greek yogurt
    2. 1/2 cup frozen mixed berries
    3. 1/2 banana
    4. 1/4 cup spinach leaves
    5. 1/2 cup almond milk (or any preferred milk)
    6. 1 scoop protein powder (optional)
- Instructions:
    1. Combine all ingredients in a blender.
    2. Blend until smooth and creamy.
    3. If the smoothie is too thick, add more milk until desired consistency is reached.

4. Pour into a glass and enjoy!

LUNCH RECIPES

Quinoa Salad with Grilled Chicken:

- Ingredients:
    1. 1/2 cup quinoa, rinsed
    2. 1 cup water or low-sodium chicken broth
    3. 1 grilled chicken breast, sliced
    4. 1/4 cup cherry tomatoes, halved
    5. 1/4 cup cucumber, diced

6. 2 tablespoons feta cheese, crumbled
7. 1 tablespoon olive oil
8. 1 tablespoon lemon juice
9. Salt and pepper to taste
- Instructions:
    1. In a saucepan, bring water or chicken broth to a boil.
    2. Add quinoa, reduce heat to low, cover, and simmer for 15-20 minutes or until quinoa is cooked and liquid is absorbed. Let it cool.
    3. In a large bowl, combine cooked quinoa, grilled chicken slices, cherry tomatoes, cucumber, and feta cheese.
    4. In a small bowl, whisk together olive oil, lemon juice, salt, and pepper to make the dressing.

5. Drizzle the dressing over the salad and toss gently to coat. Serve chilled or at room temperature.

Turkey and Avocado Wrap:

- Ingredients:
  1. 1 whole grain wrap or tortilla
  2. 3 slices deli turkey breast
  3. 1/4 avocado, sliced
  4. 1/4 cup spinach leaves
  5. 1/4 cup shredded carrots
  6. 1 tablespoon hummus
- Instructions:
  1. Lay the wrap flat on a clean surface.

2. Spread hummus evenly over the wrap.
3. Layer turkey slices, avocado slices, spinach leaves, and shredded carrots on top of the hummus.
4. Roll the wrap tightly, folding in the sides as you go.
5. Slice the wrap in half diagonally and serve.

Salmon and Quinoa Bowl:

- Ingredients:
    1. 1/2 cup cooked quinoa

2. 4 oz grilled or baked salmon fillet, flaked
  3. 1/4 cup steamed broccoli florets
  4. 1/4 cup sliced bell peppers (any color)
  5. 1 tablespoon sesame seeds
  6. 1 tablespoon soy sauce or tamari
  7. 1 teaspoon honey
  8. 1 teaspoon rice vinegar
- Instructions:
  1. Arrange cooked quinoa in a bowl.
  2. Top with flaked salmon, steamed broccoli, and sliced bell peppers.
  3. In a small bowl, whisk together soy sauce, honey, and rice vinegar to make the dressing.
  4. Drizzle the dressing over the bowl.

5. Sprinkle sesame seeds on top and serve.

Vegetable and Lentil Soup:

- Ingredients:
    1. 1/2 cup dried green lentils, rinsed
    2. 4 cups low-sodium vegetable broth
    3. 1 cup mixed vegetables (carrots, celery, onion, bell peppers)
    4. 2 cloves garlic, minced
    5. 1 teaspoon dried thyme
    6. Salt and pepper to taste
- Instructions:

1. In a large pot, combine vegetable broth, lentils, mixed vegetables, garlic, and thyme.
2. Bring to a boil, then reduce heat to low and simmer for 20-25 minutes or until lentils are tender.
3. Season with salt and pepper to taste.
4. Serve hot, optionally garnished with fresh herbs like parsley or cilantro.

Caprese Salad with Whole Grain Bread:

- Ingredients:
    1. 1 large tomato, sliced

2. 4 oz fresh mozzarella cheese, sliced
3. Fresh basil leaves
4. 1 tablespoon balsamic glaze
5. 2 slices whole grain bread, toasted
6. 1 tablespoon olive oil
7. Salt and pepper to taste
- Instructions:
    1. Arrange tomato slices and mozzarella slices on a plate, alternating with basil leaves.
    2. Drizzle balsamic glaze over the salad.
    3. Season with salt and pepper.
    4. Serve with toasted whole grain bread drizzled with olive oil.

DINNER RECIPES

Baked Lemon Herb Chicken with Roasted Vegetables:

- Ingredients:
    1. 2 boneless, skinless chicken breasts
    2. 1 lemon, sliced
    3. 2 cloves garlic, minced
    4. 1 teaspoon dried thyme
    5. 1 teaspoon dried rosemary
    6. Salt and pepper to taste
    7. 2 cups mixed vegetables (such as carrots, broccoli, bell peppers)
    8. 1 tablespoon olive oil
- Instructions:
    1. Preheat the oven to 375°F (190°C).

2. Place chicken breasts in a baking dish and season with minced garlic, dried thyme, dried rosemary, salt, and pepper.
3. Arrange lemon slices on top of the chicken.
4. In a separate bowl, toss mixed vegetables with olive oil, salt, and pepper.
5. Place the seasoned vegetables around the chicken in the baking dish.
6. Bake for 25-30 minutes or until the chicken is cooked through and the vegetables are tender. Serve hot.

Vegetable Stir-Fry with Tofu:

- Ingredients:
    1. 1 block extra firm tofu, pressed and cubed
    2. 2 cups mixed vegetables (such as bell peppers, broccoli, carrots, snap peas)
    3. 2 cloves garlic, minced
    4. 2 tablespoons soy sauce or tamari
    5. 1 tablespoon sesame oil
    6. 1 tablespoon rice vinegar
    7. Cooked brown rice or quinoa for serving
    8. Sesame seeds for garnish (optional)
- Instructions:
    1. Heat sesame oil in a large skillet or wok over medium-high heat.

2. Add cubed tofu to the skillet and cook until golden brown on all sides, about 5-7 minutes. Remove from the skillet and set aside.
3. In the same skillet, add minced garlic and mixed vegetables. Stir-fry for 3-4 minutes until vegetables are tender-crisp.
4. Return the cooked tofu to the skillet.
5. Add soy sauce and rice vinegar to the skillet, tossing everything together until evenly coated.
6. Serve the stir-fry hot over cooked brown rice or quinoa. Garnish with sesame seeds if desired.

Salmon with Asparagus and Lemon Dill Sauce:

- Ingredients:
  1. 2 salmon fillets
  2. 1 bunch asparagus, trimmed
  3. 1 lemon, sliced
  4. Salt and pepper to taste
  5. 2 tablespoons chopped fresh dill
  6. 1/4 cup Greek yogurt
  7. 1 tablespoon Dijon mustard
- Instructions:
  1. Preheat the oven to 400°F (200°C).
  2. Place salmon fillets on a baking sheet lined with parchment paper. Season with salt, pepper, and half of the chopped dill. Top

each fillet with lemon slices.
3. Arrange asparagus around the salmon on the baking sheet. Drizzle with olive oil and season with salt and pepper.
4. Bake for 12-15 minutes or until the salmon is cooked through and the asparagus is tender.
5. In a small bowl, whisk together Greek yogurt, Dijon mustard, remaining chopped dill, and lemon juice.
6. Serve the baked salmon and asparagus hot, drizzled with the lemon dill sauce.

Turkey and Vegetable Skillet:

- Ingredients:
    1. 1 lb ground turkey
    2. 1 onion, diced
    3. 2 cloves garlic, minced
    4. 1 bell pepper, diced
    5. 1 zucchini, diced
    6. 1 cup cherry tomatoes, halved
    7. 1 teaspoon dried oregano
    8. 1 teaspoon paprika
    9. Salt and pepper to taste
    10. 2 tablespoons olive oil
- Instructions:
    1. Heat olive oil in a large skillet over medium heat.
    2. Add diced onion and minced garlic to the skillet, sauté until fragrant.
    3. Add ground turkey to the skillet, breaking it up with

a spoon, and cook until browned.
4. Stir in diced bell pepper, zucchini, cherry tomatoes, dried oregano, paprika, salt, and pepper.
5. Cook for 8-10 minutes, stirring occasionally, until vegetables are tender and tomatoes are softened.
6. Serve hot, optionally garnished with fresh herbs like parsley or basil.

Vegetable and Bean Soup:

- Ingredients:
    1. 1 tablespoon olive oil

2. 1 onion, diced
3. 2 carrots, diced
4. 2 celery stalks, diced
5. 2 cloves garlic, minced
6. 1 can (15 oz) white beans, drained and rinsed
7. 4 cups low-sodium vegetable broth
8. 1 can (14.5 oz) diced tomatoes
9. 1 teaspoon dried thyme
10. Salt and pepper to taste

- Instructions:
    1. Heat olive oil in a large pot over medium heat.
    2. Add diced onion, carrots, and celery to the pot. Sauté until vegetables are softened.
    3. Add minced garlic and cook for another minute until fragrant.
    4. Stir in white beans, vegetable broth, diced

tomatoes (with juices), dried thyme, salt, and pepper.
5. Bring the soup to a boil, then reduce heat to low and simmer for 15-20 minutes.

6. Taste and adjust seasoning if needed. Serve hot, optionally garnished with freshly chopped parsley.

APPETIZER RECIPES

Vegetable Crudité with Hummus:

- Ingredients:
    1. Assorted raw vegetables (carrots, celery, bell peppers, cucumber, cherry tomatoes)

            2. Hummus (store-bought or homemade)
    - Instructions:
        1. Wash and prepare the raw vegetables by cutting them into bite-sized sticks or slices.
        2. Arrange the vegetable sticks on a serving platter.
        3. Place a bowl of hummus in the center of the platter.
        4. Serve the vegetable crudité with hummus for dipping.

Caprese Skewers:

    - Ingredients:
        1. Cherry tomatoes

2. Fresh mozzarella cheese, cut into cubes
3. Fresh basil leaves
4. Balsamic glaze (store-bought or homemade)
5. Toothpicks or skewers
- Instructions:
    1. Thread one cherry tomato, one cube of mozzarella cheese, and one basil leaf onto each toothpick or skewer.
    2. Arrange the caprese skewers on a serving platter.
    3. Drizzle balsamic glaze over the skewers just before serving.

Guacamole with Baked Tortilla Chips:

- Ingredients:
    1. 2 ripe avocados
    2. 1 small tomato, diced
    3. 1/4 cup red onion, finely chopped
    4. 1 clove garlic, minced
    5. 1 lime, juiced
    6. Salt and pepper to taste
    7. Baked whole grain tortilla chips (store-bought or homemade)
- Instructions:
    1. Cut the avocados in half, remove the pits, and scoop the flesh into a bowl.
    2. Mash the avocado with a fork until smooth or leave it slightly chunky if desired.

3. Stir in diced tomato, chopped red onion, minced garlic, and lime juice.
4. Season with salt and pepper to taste.
5. Serve the guacamole with baked whole grain tortilla chips for dipping.

Smoked Salmon Cucumber Bites:

- Ingredients:
    1. English cucumber, sliced into rounds
    2. Smoked salmon slices
    3. Cream cheese
    4. Fresh dill, for garnish

- Instructions:
    1. Lay cucumber slices on a serving platter.
    2. Spread a small amount of cream cheese on each cucumber slice.
    3. Top with a piece of smoked salmon.
    4. Garnish with fresh dill.
    5. Secure with toothpicks if necessary and serve chilled.

Stuffed Mushrooms:

- Ingredients:

1. Large white mushrooms, cleaned with stems removed
2. 1/2 cup cream cheese, softened
3. 1/4 cup grated Parmesan cheese
4. 2 tablespoons chopped fresh parsley
5. 1 clove garlic, minced
6. Salt and pepper to taste
7. Olive oil

- Instructions:
    1. Preheat the oven to 375°F (190°C).
    2. In a bowl, mix together softened cream cheese, grated Parmesan cheese, chopped parsley, minced garlic, salt, and pepper until well combined.
    3. Stuff each mushroom cap with the cream cheese mixture.

4. Place stuffed mushrooms on a baking sheet lined with parchment paper.
5. Drizzle with olive oil and bake for 15-20 minutes or until mushrooms are tender and filling is golden brown.
6. Serve hot, optionally garnished with additional chopped parsley.

HEALTHY RECIPES

Salmon Salad with Lemon-Dill Dressing:

- Ingredients:
    1. 4 oz grilled or baked salmon fillet, flaked
    2. Mixed salad greens (lettuce, spinach, arugula)
    3. 1/4 cup cherry tomatoes, halved
    4. 1/4 cucumber, sliced
    5. 1/4 red onion, thinly sliced
    6. 1 tablespoon chopped fresh dill
    7. 1 tablespoon olive oil
    8. 1 tablespoon lemon juice
    9. Salt and pepper to taste
- Instructions:
    1. In a large bowl, combine mixed salad greens, cherry

tomatoes, cucumber slices, and thinly sliced red onion.
2. Top the salad with flaked salmon.
3. In a small bowl, whisk together olive oil, lemon juice, chopped dill, salt, and pepper to make the dressing.
4. Drizzle the dressing over the salad and toss gently to coat. Serve immediately.

Quinoa and Black Bean Salad:

- Ingredients:
    1. 1/2 cup quinoa, rinsed

2. 1 cup water or low-sodium vegetable broth
3. 1 can (15 oz) black beans, drained and rinsed
4. 1/2 cup corn kernels (fresh or frozen)
5. 1/4 cup diced red bell pepper
6. 1/4 cup chopped fresh cilantro
7. 2 tablespoons lime juice
8. 1 tablespoon olive oil
9. 1 teaspoon ground cumin
10. Salt and pepper to taste

- Instructions:
    1. In a saucepan, bring water or vegetable broth to a boil. Add quinoa, reduce heat to low, cover, and simmer for 15-20 minutes or until quinoa is cooked and liquid is absorbed. Let it cool.

2. In a large bowl, combine cooked quinoa, black beans, corn kernels, diced red bell pepper, and chopped cilantro.
3. In a small bowl, whisk together lime juice, olive oil, ground cumin, salt, and pepper to make the dressing.
4. Drizzle the dressing over the quinoa salad and toss gently to combine. Serve chilled or at room temperature.

Turkey and Vegetable Stir-Fry:

- Ingredients:
    1. 1 lb ground turkey
    2. 2 cups mixed vegetables (such as broccoli, bell peppers, carrots, snap peas)
    3. 2 cloves garlic, minced
    4. 2 tablespoons low-sodium soy sauce or tamari
    5. 1 tablespoon sesame oil
    6. 1 tablespoon rice vinegar
    7. Cooked brown rice for serving
- Instructions:
    1. Heat sesame oil in a large skillet or wok over medium-high heat.
    2. Add minced garlic and ground turkey to the skillet. Cook until turkey is

browned and cooked through.
3. Add mixed vegetables to the skillet and stir-fry for 3-4 minutes until vegetables are tender-crisp.
4. In a small bowl, whisk together soy sauce and rice vinegar. Pour the sauce over the turkey and vegetables, tossing to coat.
5. Serve the turkey and vegetable stir-fry hot over cooked brown rice.

Spinach and Chickpea Curry:

- Ingredients:
    1. 1 tablespoon olive oil
    2. 1 onion, diced
    3. 2 cloves garlic, minced
    4. 1 tablespoon grated ginger
    5. 1 tablespoon curry powder
    6. 1 teaspoon ground cumin
    7. 1 can (15 oz) chickpeas, drained and rinsed
    8. 2 cups chopped fresh spinach
    9. 1 can (14.5 oz) diced tomatoes
    10. 1/2 cup coconut milk
    11. Salt and pepper to taste
- Instructions:
    1. Heat olive oil in a large skillet over medium heat.
    2. Add diced onion, minced garlic, and grated ginger to

the skillet. Sauté until onion is soft and translucent.
3. Stir in curry powder and ground cumin, cooking for 1-2 minutes until fragrant.
4. Add chickpeas, chopped spinach, diced tomatoes (with juices), and coconut milk to the skillet. Season with salt and pepper.
5. Simmer for 10-15 minutes, stirring occasionally, until the sauce has thickened slightly and the spinach is wilted.
6. Serve the spinach and chickpea curry hot, optionally garnished with chopped cilantro, and accompanied by cooked brown rice or whole wheat naan.

Vegetable and Lentil Soup:

- Ingredients:
    1. 1 tablespoon olive oil
    2. 1 onion, diced
    3. 2 carrots, diced
    4. 2 celery stalks, diced
    5. 2 cloves garlic, minced
    6. 1 cup dried green lentils, rinsed
    7. 4 cups low-sodium vegetable broth
    8. 1 can (14.5 oz) diced tomatoes
    9. 1 teaspoon dried thyme
    10. Salt and pepper to taste
- Instructions:
    1. Heat olive oil in a large pot over medium heat.
    2. Add diced onion, carrots, and celery to the pot. Sauté

until vegetables are softened.
3. Add minced garlic and cook for another minute until fragrant.
4. Stir in dried green lentils, vegetable broth, diced tomatoes (with juices), dried thyme, salt, and pepper.
5. Bring the soup to a boil, then reduce heat to low and simmer for 20-25 minutes or until lentils are tender.
6. Taste and adjust seasoning if needed. Serve hot, optionally garnished with freshly chopped parsley.

SNACKS AND DESSERT RECIPES

SNACKS:

Yogurt with Berries and Almonds:

- Ingredients:
    1. 1/2 cup Greek yogurt
    2. 1/4 cup mixed berries (such as blueberries, raspberries, strawberries)
    3. 1 tablespoon sliced almonds
    4. 1 teaspoon honey (optional)
- Instructions:
    1. Spoon Greek yogurt into a bowl.
    2. Top with mixed berries and sliced almonds.

3. Drizzle with honey if desired.

Vegetable Sticks with Hummus:

- Ingredients:
    1. Assorted raw vegetable sticks (carrots, celery, bell peppers)
    2. Hummus (store-bought or homemade)
- Instructions:
    1. Wash and prepare the raw vegetables by cutting them into sticks.
    2. Serve with hummus for dipping.

Apple Slices with Peanut Butter:

- Ingredients:
    1. 1 apple, sliced
    2. 2 tablespoons peanut butter (or almond butter)
- Instructions:
    1. Spread peanut butter on apple slices.
    2. Enjoy as a crunchy and satisfying snack.

Cottage Cheese with Pineapple:

- Ingredients:

    1. 1/2 cup low-fat cottage cheese
    2. 1/4 cup diced pineapple (fresh or canned in juice)
- Instructions:
    1. Place cottage cheese in a bowl.
    2. Top with diced pineapple.

Trail Mix:

- Ingredients:
    1. 1/4 cup mixed nuts (almonds, walnuts, cashews)
    2. 2 tablespoons dried fruit (raisins, cranberries, apricots)

3. 1 tablespoon dark chocolate chips or chunks
   - Instructions:
      1. Mix all ingredients together in a bowl.
      2. Portion out into small snack-sized bags for convenience.

DESSERTS:

Frozen Yogurt Bark:

   - Ingredients:
      1. 1 cup Greek yogurt
      2. 1 tablespoon honey or maple syrup

3. 1/4 cup mixed berries (such as blueberries, raspberries, strawberries)
4. 2 tablespoons granola
- Instructions:
  1. Line a baking sheet with parchment paper.
  2. In a bowl, mix Greek yogurt with honey or maple syrup.
  3. Spread the yogurt mixture onto the parchment paper in an even layer.
  4. Sprinkle mixed berries and granola evenly over the yogurt.
  5. Freeze for 2-3 hours until firm, then break into pieces and enjoy.

Banana Oatmeal Cookies:

- Ingredients:
    1. 2 ripe bananas, mashed
    2. 1 cup rolled oats
    3. 1/4 cup chopped nuts (such as walnuts or almonds)
    4. 1/4 cup dark chocolate chips (optional)
    5. 1 teaspoon cinnamon
- Instructions:
    1. Preheat the oven to 350°F (175°C) and line a baking sheet with parchment paper.
    2. In a bowl, combine mashed bananas, rolled oats, chopped nuts, dark chocolate chips (if using), and cinnamon. Mix until well combined.

3. Drop spoonfuls of the mixture onto the prepared baking sheet and flatten slightly with the back of a spoon.
4. Bake for 15-20 minutes or until cookies are golden brown.
5. Allow to cool before serving.

Chia Seed Pudding:

- Ingredients:
    1. 1/4 cup chia seeds
    2. 1 cup almond milk (or any preferred milk)

3. 1 tablespoon honey or maple syrup
4. 1/2 teaspoon vanilla extract
5. Fresh fruit for topping (such as sliced strawberries, kiwi, or mango)
- Instructions:
    1. In a bowl, whisk together chia seeds, almond milk, honey or maple syrup, and vanilla extract.
    2. Cover and refrigerate for at least 2 hours or overnight, until the mixture thickens into a pudding-like consistency.
    3. Serve topped with fresh fruit.

Baked Apples with Cinnamon and Walnuts:

- Ingredients:
    1. 2 apples, cored
    2. 2 tablespoons chopped walnuts
    3. 1 tablespoon honey or maple syrup
    4. 1/2 teaspoon cinnamon
    5. 1/4 cup water
- Instructions:
    1. Preheat the oven to 375°F (190°C).
    2. In a small bowl, mix chopped walnuts, honey or maple syrup, and cinnamon.
    3. Stuff each cored apple with the walnut mixture.
    4. Place stuffed apples in a baking dish and pour

water into the bottom of the dish.
5. Bake for 25-30 minutes or until apples are tender.
6. Serve warm.

Frozen Banana Bites:

- Ingredients:
    1. 2 ripe bananas, peeled and cut into chunks
    2. 1/4 cup peanut butter (or almond butter)
    3. 1/4 cup dark chocolate chips
    4. 2 tablespoons chopped nuts (such as almonds or peanuts)

- Instructions:
    1. Line a baking sheet with parchment paper.
    2. Spread peanut butter on banana chunks and sandwich them together.
    3. Place banana sandwiches on the prepared baking sheet and freeze for 1-2 hours until firm.
    4. Melt dark chocolate chips in a microwave-safe bowl in 30-second intervals, stirring until smooth.
    5. Dip frozen banana sandwiches halfway into the melted chocolate, then sprinkle with chopped nuts.
    6. Place back on the baking sheet and freeze for an additional 30 minutes until chocolate is set. Enjoy!

28DAY MEAL PLAN

Day 1:

- Breakfast: Oatmeal with Berries (oats cooked in water or milk topped with mixed berries)
- Lunch: Turkey and Avocado Wrap (whole grain wrap filled with deli turkey breast, avocado slices, spinach leaves, shredded carrots, and hummus)
- Dinner: Baked Lemon Herb Chicken with Roasted Vegetables (chicken breast seasoned with lemon, garlic, thyme, and rosemary, served with a side of roasted mixed vegetables)

Day 2:

- Breakfast: Greek Yogurt Parfait (Greek yogurt layered with granola and mixed fruits)
- Lunch: Vegetable and Lentil Soup (homemade soup with green lentils, carrots, celery, onion, garlic, and vegetable broth)
- Dinner: Salmon with Asparagus and Lemon Dill Sauce (grilled or baked salmon fillet with steamed asparagus, topped with a lemon dill sauce)

Day 3:

- Breakfast: Spinach and Tomato Omelette (eggs filled with spinach, tomatoes, and feta cheese)

- Lunch: Caprese Salad with Whole Grain Bread (sliced tomatoes, fresh mozzarella, and basil drizzled with balsamic glaze, served with whole grain bread)
- Dinner: Vegetable and Chickpea Stir-Fry (stir-fried mixed vegetables and chickpeas in a sesame ginger sauce, served over brown rice)

Day 4:

- Breakfast: Smoothie with Protein (blend Greek yogurt, mixed berries, banana, spinach, almond milk, and protein powder)
- Lunch: Quinoa Salad with Grilled Chicken (quinoa mixed with grilled chicken, cherry tomatoes, cucumber, feta cheese, and a lemon herb dressing)

- Dinner: Turkey Meatballs with Marinara Sauce and Zucchini Noodles (baked turkey meatballs served with zucchini noodles and marinara sauce)

Day 5:

- Breakfast: Avocado Toast with Egg (whole grain toast topped with mashed avocado and a fried or poached egg)
- Lunch: Greek Salad with Grilled Shrimp (mixed greens, cucumber, cherry tomatoes, red onion, feta cheese, olives, and grilled shrimp with a Greek vinaigrette)
- Dinner: Lentil and Vegetable Curry (curried lentils with mixed vegetables served over brown rice)

Day 6:

- Breakfast: Cottage Cheese with Pineapple (low-fat cottage cheese topped with diced pineapple)
- Lunch: Chicken Caesar Salad (grilled chicken breast, romaine lettuce, cherry tomatoes, croutons, and Caesar dressing)
- Dinner: Beef and Broccoli Stir-Fry (stir-fried beef strips and broccoli florets in a garlic ginger sauce, served over quinoa)

Day 7:

- Breakfast: Banana Oatmeal Cookies (homemade cookies made with mashed bananas, oats, nuts, and cinnamon)

- Lunch: Vegetable and Tofu Stir-Fry (stir-fried tofu and mixed vegetables in a teriyaki sauce, served over brown rice)
- Dinner: Stuffed Bell Peppers with Quinoa and Black Beans (bell peppers stuffed with quinoa, black beans, corn, tomatoes, and spices, baked until tender)

Day 8:

- Breakfast: Greek Yogurt with Berries and Almonds (Greek yogurt topped with mixed berries and sliced almonds)
- Lunch: Turkey and Vegetable Skillet (ground turkey cooked with mixed vegetables, seasoned with herbs and spices)
- Dinner: Baked Salmon with Steamed Broccoli and Quinoa (salmon fillet

baked with lemon and herbs, served with steamed broccoli and quinoa)

Day 9:

- Breakfast: Spinach and Feta Breakfast Wrap (whole grain wrap filled with scrambled eggs, sautéed spinach, and crumbled feta cheese)
- Lunch: Lentil Soup with Whole Grain Bread (homemade lentil soup served with whole grain bread)
- Dinner: Chicken and Vegetable Stir-Fry (sliced chicken breast stir-fried with mixed vegetables in a light soy sauce, served over brown rice)

Day 10:

- Breakfast: Banana Smoothie with Peanut Butter (blend banana, Greek yogurt, almond milk, spinach, and peanut butter)
- Lunch: Caprese Quinoa Salad (quinoa mixed with cherry tomatoes, fresh mozzarella, basil, and balsamic glaze)
- Dinner: Vegetable and Bean Enchiladas (baked enchiladas filled with mixed vegetables, black beans, and cheese, topped with salsa)

Day 11:

- Breakfast: Whole Grain Pancakes with Mixed Berries (whole grain pancakes topped with mixed berries and a drizzle of honey)

- Lunch: Tuna Salad Sandwich on Whole Grain Bread (tuna salad made with Greek yogurt, served on whole grain bread with lettuce and tomato)
- Dinner: Grilled Chicken with Roasted Sweet Potatoes and Green Beans (grilled chicken breast served with roasted sweet potatoes and steamed green beans)

Day 12:

- Breakfast: Veggie Omelette with Whole Wheat Toast (omelette filled with sautéed vegetables, served with whole wheat toast)
- Lunch: Quinoa and Black Bean Salad (quinoa salad with black beans, corn, bell peppers, and cilantro lime dressing)
- Dinner: Beef and Vegetable Stir-Fry with Brown Rice (sliced beef stir-fried

with mixed vegetables in a ginger garlic sauce, served over brown rice)

Day 13:

- Breakfast: Overnight Oats with Almond Butter and Banana (oats soaked overnight in almond milk, topped with almond butter and sliced banana)
- Lunch: Mediterranean Chickpea Salad (chickpea salad with cucumber, tomatoes, olives, feta cheese, and lemon herb dressing)
- Dinner: Shrimp and Vegetable Skewers with Quinoa (grilled shrimp and mixed vegetables served on skewers, accompanied by quinoa)

Day 14:

- Breakfast: Greek Yogurt Parfait with Granola and Honey (Greek yogurt layered with granola and drizzled with honey)
- Lunch: Chicken Caesar Wrap (grilled chicken, romaine lettuce, Parmesan cheese, and Caesar dressing wrapped in a whole grain tortilla)
- Dinner: Lentil and Spinach Curry with Brown Rice (curried lentils and spinach served over brown rice)

Day 15:

- Breakfast: Scrambled Eggs with Spinach and Tomatoes (scrambled eggs cooked with sautéed spinach and diced tomatoes)

- Lunch: Turkey and Avocado Salad (sliced turkey breast, mixed greens, avocado slices, cherry tomatoes, and balsamic vinaigrette)
- Dinner: Baked Cod with Roasted Vegetables (cod fillets seasoned with herbs and lemon, served with roasted vegetables)

Day 16:

- Breakfast: Greek Yogurt with Mixed Berries and Almonds (Greek yogurt topped with mixed berries and sliced almonds)
- Lunch: Quinoa and Vegetable Buddha Bowl (quinoa, roasted vegetables, chickpeas, avocado slices, and tahini dressing)
- Dinner: Chicken and Vegetable Stir-Fry with Brown Rice (sliced chicken breast stir-fried with mixed

vegetables in a teriyaki sauce, served over brown rice)

Day 17:

- Breakfast: Whole Grain Toast with Peanut Butter and Banana Slices (whole grain toast topped with peanut butter and sliced banana)
- Lunch: Mediterranean Chickpea Wrap (whole grain wrap filled with chickpeas, cucumber, tomatoes, feta cheese, and Greek yogurt dressing)
- Dinner: Beef and Broccoli Stir-Fry with Quinoa (sliced beef stir-fried with broccoli florets in a garlic ginger sauce, served over quinoa)

Day 18:

- Breakfast: Smoothie Bowl with Mixed Berries and Granola (smoothie bowl blended with mixed berries, topped with granola, and sliced fruit)
- Lunch: Lentil Soup with Whole Grain Bread (homemade lentil soup served with whole grain bread)
- Dinner: Grilled Salmon with Steamed Asparagus and Sweet Potatoes (grilled salmon fillets served with steamed asparagus and roasted sweet potatoes)

Day 19:

- Breakfast: Vegetable Omelette with Feta Cheese (omelette filled with sautéed vegetables and crumbled feta cheese)

- Lunch: Greek Salad with Grilled Chicken (mixed greens, cucumber, cherry tomatoes, red onion, feta cheese, olives, grilled chicken, and Greek vinaigrette)
- Dinner: Turkey Meatballs with Marinara Sauce and Zucchini Noodles (baked turkey meatballs served with zucchini noodles and marinara sauce)

Day 20:

- Breakfast: Overnight Oats with Almond Butter and Chia Seeds (overnight oats soaked in almond milk, topped with almond butter and chia seeds)
- Lunch: Tuna Salad Stuffed Avocado (tuna salad made with Greek yogurt, served in halved avocados)

- Dinner: Vegetable and Chickpea Curry with Brown Rice (curried vegetables and chickpeas served over brown rice)

Day 21:

- Breakfast: Whole Grain Pancakes with Mixed Berries and Maple Syrup (whole grain pancakes topped with mixed berries and a drizzle of maple syrup)
- Lunch: Caprese Salad with Whole Grain Bread (sliced tomatoes, fresh mozzarella, basil, balsamic glaze, and whole grain bread)
- Dinner: Stuffed Bell Peppers with Quinoa and Black Beans (bell peppers stuffed with quinoa, black beans, corn, tomatoes, and spices, baked until tender)

Day 22:

- Breakfast: Scrambled Eggs with Spinach and Mushrooms (scrambled eggs cooked with sautéed spinach and mushrooms)
- Lunch: Turkey and Cranberry Wrap (sliced turkey breast, cranberry sauce, mixed greens, and cream cheese in a whole grain wrap)
- Dinner: Baked Chicken with Roasted Brussels Sprouts and Sweet Potatoes (chicken breasts baked with herbs, served with roasted Brussels sprouts and sweet potatoes)

Day 23:

- Breakfast: Greek Yogurt with Honey and Walnuts (Greek yogurt topped with honey and chopped walnuts)
- Lunch: Quinoa Salad with Grilled Vegetables (quinoa mixed with grilled vegetables, feta cheese, and balsamic vinaigrette)
- Dinner: Grilled Fish Tacos with Cabbage Slaw (grilled fish fillets served in corn tortillas with cabbage slaw and avocado)

Day 24:

- Breakfast: Whole Grain Toast with Avocado and Tomato Slices (whole grain toast topped with mashed avocado and sliced tomatoes)

- Lunch: Chickpea and Vegetable Stir-Fry (sautéed chickpeas and mixed vegetables in a teriyaki sauce, served over brown rice)
- Dinner: Beef and Broccoli Stir-Fry with Quinoa (sliced beef stir-fried with broccoli florets in a garlic ginger sauce, served over quinoa)

Day 25:

- Breakfast: Smoothie with Mixed Berries and Spinach (smoothie blended with mixed berries, spinach, Greek yogurt, and almond milk)
- Lunch: Mediterranean Salad with Grilled Chicken (mixed greens, cucumber, cherry tomatoes, olives, feta cheese, grilled chicken, and Greek vinaigrette)
- Dinner: Lentil and Vegetable Curry with Brown Rice (curried lentils and

mixed vegetables served over brown rice)

Day 26:

- Breakfast: Banana Oatmeal Pancakes (pancakes made with mashed bananas, oats, and eggs, served with maple syrup)
- Lunch: Caprese Sandwich with Whole Grain Bread (sliced tomatoes, fresh mozzarella, basil, balsamic glaze, and whole grain bread)
- Dinner: Turkey Chili with Cornbread Muffins (homemade turkey chili served with cornbread muffins)

Day 27:

- Breakfast: Veggie Breakfast Burrito (whole grain tortilla filled with scrambled eggs, sautéed vegetables, and salsa)
- Lunch: Greek Quinoa Bowl (quinoa topped with chickpeas, cucumber, tomatoes, olives, feta cheese, and Greek yogurt dressing)
- Dinner: Baked Salmon with Roasted Vegetables and Quinoa (salmon fillets baked with lemon and herbs, served with roasted vegetables and quinoa)

Day 28:

- Breakfast: Overnight Chia Seed Pudding with Mixed Berries (chia seed

- pudding soaked in almond milk, topped with mixed berries)
- Lunch: Tuna Salad Stuffed Tomatoes (tuna salad made with Greek yogurt, served in halved tomatoes)
- Dinner: Vegetable and Bean Enchiladas with Salad (baked enchiladas filled with mixed vegetables, black beans, and cheese, served with a side salad)

CONCLUSION

"Congratulations on taking the first step towards breathing easier and living better! With this cookbook, you've gained a powerful tool to help manage your COPD and improve your overall health.

Remember, every delicious bite and nourishing meal is a step towards a healthier, happier you. Don't let COPD hold you back - take control of your diet, your breathing, and your life.

You got this! And with this cookbook by your side, you'll be cooking up a storm and breathing easy in no time. Happy cooking, and happy healing!"

This conclusion aims to:

- Congratulate the reader on taking the first step towards managing their COPD
- Emphasize the importance of diet in managing COPD
- Encourage the reader to take control of their health and well-being
- End with a positive and uplifting note, wishing the reader happy cooking and happy healing.

THE END

www.ingramcontent.com/pod-product-compliance
Lightning Source LLC
Chambersburg PA
CBHW050114230526
45470CB00004B/1831